THE
Panic
Button
BOOK

Relieve stress and anxiety whenever they strike

TAMMI KIRKNESS

Houghton Mifflin Harcourt
Boston • New York • 2020

This book is dedicated to the
one in four people who will
experience anxiety in their lives.

My wish is that you recognize how magnificent
your brain is, how much bravery your heart holds,
and that you get to experience what it feels like
to go with the flow.

This book is also dedicated to
all the people who know and love
these courageous individuals.

I wish you a lifetime of compassion,
inner strength, and the confidence
to support those around you.

Introduction

For as long as I can remember I was an overthinker, over-analyzer, and perfectionist. It turns out that these attributes formed part of something referred to as high-functioning anxiety. I was a master at striving for results, feeding off recognition, and looking like I was blitzing life—all the while running on a nervous energy that simply wouldn't shift.

When I was single, it was easy for me to hide my symptoms and my worries. If I was feeling like I couldn't breathe, I could skip after-work drinks. If I was replaying a conversation over and over in my head, I could stay in the shower until it started to abate.

But then I got into a relationship with a beautiful man whom I eventually moved in with and then married. Once I had someone around all the time, I couldn't hide in quite the same way. If I was close to hyperventilating, he would notice. If I got teary because I was struggling to pick what to wear to a casual lunch, he'd ask questions.

It culminated one day when I had a very teary—couldn't breathe, couldn't move my body—panic attack and he didn't know what to do. He looked terrified and I hated that. I was stuck on one of our kitchen stools with tears running down my face, completely incapacitated, and I was trying to send him mental messages on what to do. My brain was screaming at him to cover me in a heavy blanket. To not take his hand off my arm. To not try to lie me down. To play my favorite calming song. To help me to breathe. To not expect me to use the tissue he'd given me because my arms had forgotten how to move. That if he thought it was a good idea to relocate me from the kitchen stool, he'd have to carry me.

I wished for a "normal" version of myself standing close by, to walk us both through what I needed. I felt awful that he felt so helpless.

A few weeks later, when I was in a much calmer headspace, I wrote down all the scenarios that related to my anxiety and created a set of instructions that I could pick up if I felt panicky or worried.

Essentially, I created this book.

I knew that when I was feeling good I could easily instruct myself on how to keep my cool, but when I was feeling anxious, the rational part of my brain was blocked. Once I saw how much it helped me, I knew that I had to make it available for others.

Part of being a deep thinker led me to crave understanding about why people are the way they are; what makes them worry and what leads them to happiness. This curiosity steered me to a lifelong love affair with understanding people. My insatiable appetite inspired me to study psychology, yoga teaching, energy-based modalities, and coaching. I studied in ashrams, at university, with monks in the south of India; after a stint in the human resources arena, I converted this knowledge to running a life coaching and corporate wellness practice.

Anxiety comes in many flavors. Some of us have had a lifetime of secretly struggling, while looking like we're achieving our way through life. Others have talked openly about their fears and worries. Some have used medication; some haven't. But anyone who has been touched personally by anxiety can understand the stomach-twisting, leg-paralyzing, stuck-in-your-throat feeling of fear.

I believe that people with anxiety are some of the strongest, most courageous people on the planet. Despite feeling as though there's serious danger in the room, they often pull themselves together and put on a brave face.

If you are the brave person who worries all the time, I see you. I honor your efforts and hope that this book brings you a space of neutral emotions (or even positive ones) when you're feeling stuck, paralyzed, or frozen.

Begin here

Living and working

Are you feeling responsible for the world right now? Are your muscles tense? Are you struggling to switch off from work?

> **Turn to page 7**

Socializing

Are you dreading an event? Nervous about crowds? Have a difficult conversation coming up? Need to give a speech?

> **Turn to page 67**

Relationships

Are you upset with your partner? Communication breakdown? Bedroom shyness? Concerned your partner might leave you?

> **Turn to page 87**

Parenting

Are you worried you're not doing it "right"? Tired? Feeling judged? Trying to be everything to everyone?

> **Turn to page 107**

> **Resources, page 126**

Don't know where to start?
> **Start right here and turn the page**

Living & Working

Worry and anxiety will impact everybody at some point.
If you're currently experiencing fear, worry, or anxiety,
turn the page to hit the panic button and begin.

Are your muscles

feeling tense?

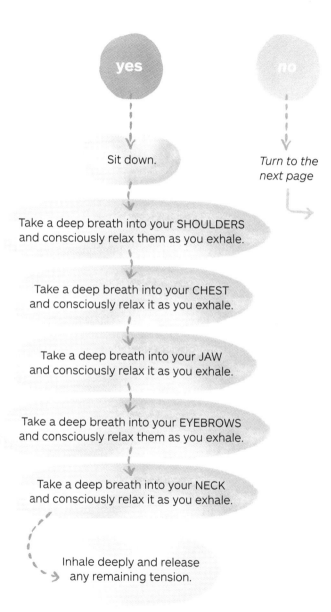

yes

no

Sit down.

Turn to the next page

Take a deep breath into your SHOULDERS and consciously relax them as you exhale.

Take a deep breath into your CHEST and consciously relax it as you exhale.

Take a deep breath into your JAW and consciously relax it as you exhale.

Take a deep breath into your EYEBROWS and consciously relax them as you exhale.

Take a deep breath into your NECK and consciously relax it as you exhale.

Inhale deeply and release any remaining tension.

Are you feeling easily startled?

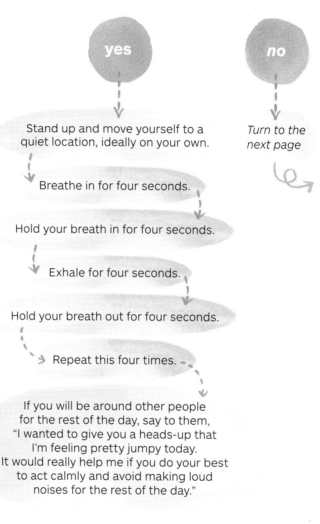

yes

no

Stand up and move yourself to a
quiet location, ideally on your own.

*Turn to the
next page*

Breathe in for four seconds.

Hold your breath in for four seconds.

Exhale for four seconds.

Hold your breath out for four seconds.

Repeat this four times.

If you will be around other people
for the rest of the day, say to them,
"I wanted to give you a heads-up that
I'm feeling pretty jumpy today.
It would really help me if you do your best
to act calmly and avoid making loud
noises for the rest of the day."

It is likely that you are experiencing hypervigilance: a feeling
of heightened alertness and edginess. This causes increased
sensitivity; for example, you may feel jumpy at loud noises or
touches to the skin. Box breathing, the technique described
here, was developed as a way to reduce these symptoms.

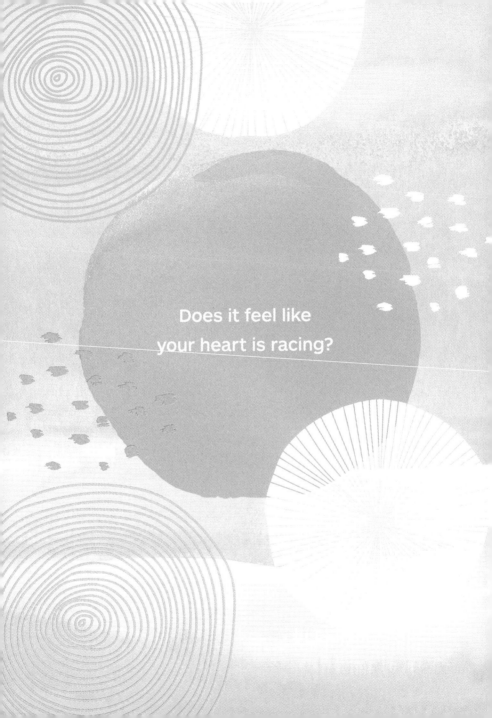

Does it feel like
your heart is racing?

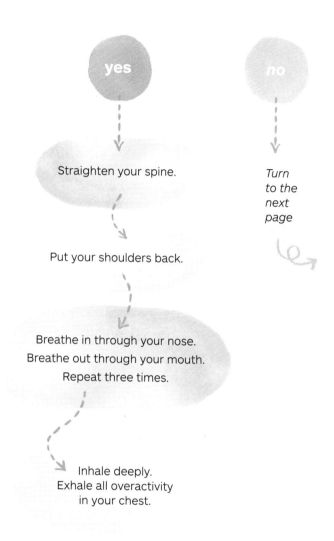

yes

no

Straighten your spine.

Turn to the next page

Put your shoulders back.

Breathe in through your nose.
Breathe out through your mouth.
Repeat three times.

Inhale deeply.
Exhale all overactivity
in your chest.

Are you worrying about something that's outside your control?

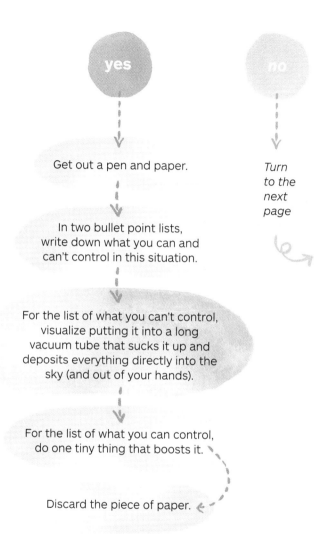

yes

no

Get out a pen and paper.

Turn to the next page

In two bullet point lists, write down what you can and can't control in this situation.

For the list of what you can't control, visualize putting it into a long vacuum tube that sucks it up and deposits everything directly into the sky (and out of your hands).

For the list of what you can control, do one tiny thing that boosts it.

Discard the piece of paper.

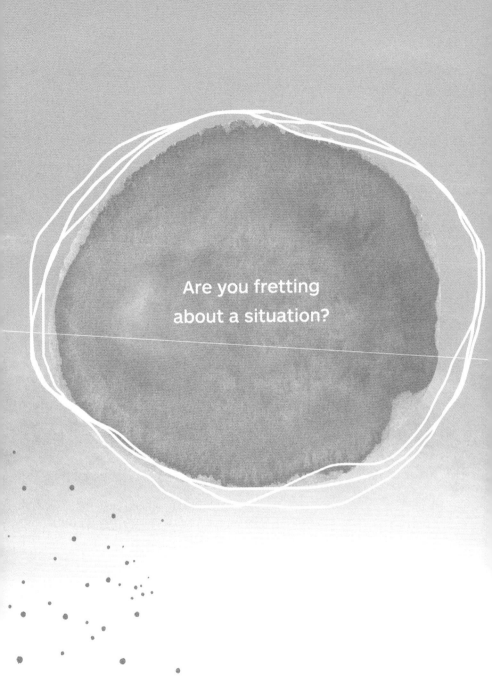

Are you fretting
about a situation?

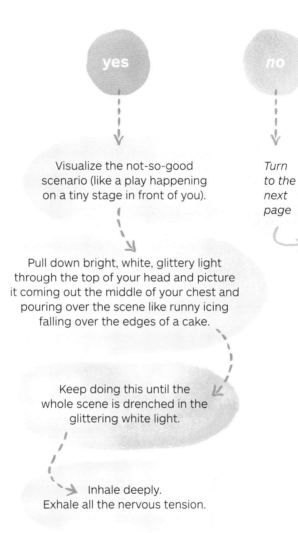

yes

no

Visualize the not-so-good scenario (like a play happening on a tiny stage in front of you).

Turn to the next page

Pull down bright, white, glittery light through the top of your head and picture it coming out the middle of your chest and pouring over the scene like runny icing falling over the edges of a cake.

Keep doing this until the whole scene is drenched in the glittering white light.

Inhale deeply.
Exhale all the nervous tension.

If the situation was a social one and you're still fretting, turn to page 67 to continue.

Are you feeling underprepared
for something?

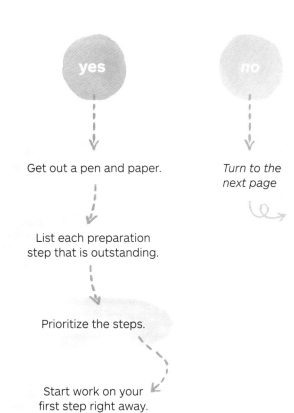

yes

no

Get out a pen and paper.

Turn to the next page

List each preparation step that is outstanding.

Prioritize the steps.

Start work on your first step right away.

Are you feeling attached
to an outcome?

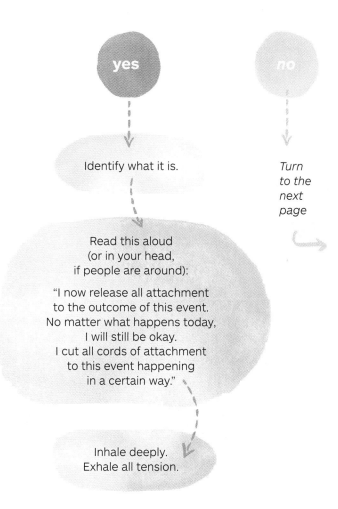

yes

no

Identify what it is.

Turn to the next page

Read this aloud
(or in your head,
if people are around):

"I now release all attachment
to the outcome of this event.
No matter what happens today,
I will still be okay.
I cut all cords of attachment
to this event happening
in a certain way."

Inhale deeply.
Exhale all tension.

When we are attached to things unfolding in a certain way, our
emotions can destabilize. The more we can release our fears of
losing something that hasn't happened yet (such as a job we've
applied for), the more okay we'll be.

Are you trying to make

something perfect?

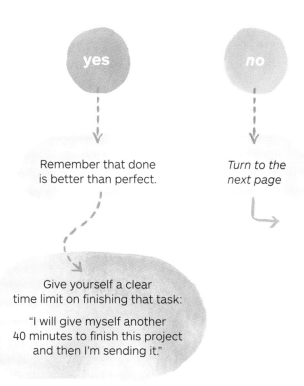

yes

Remember that done
is better than perfect.

no

*Turn to the
next page*

Give yourself a clear
time limit on finishing that task:

"I will give myself another
40 minutes to finish this project
and then I'm sending it."

Are you feeling paralyzed?

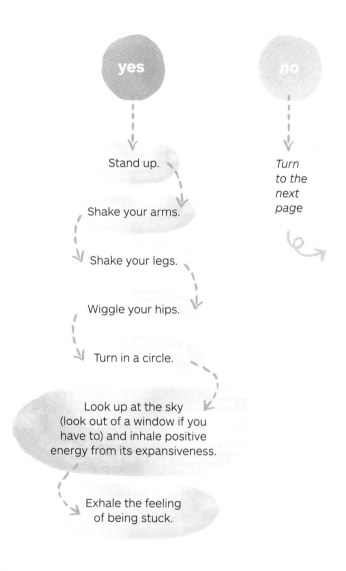

yes

no

Stand up.

Shake your arms.

Shake your legs.

Wiggle your hips.

Turn in a circle.

Look up at the sky
(look out of a window if you
have to) and inhale positive
energy from its expansiveness.

Exhale the feeling
of being stuck.

*Turn
to the
next
page*

Feeling "stuck," tense, and paralyzed are common symptoms
of anxiety.

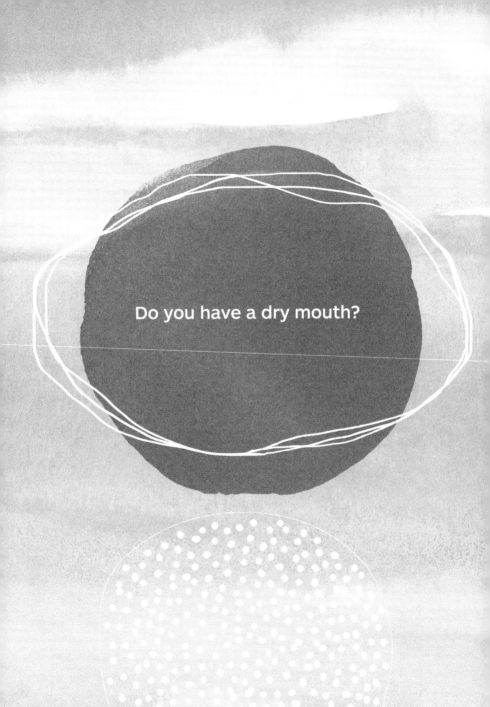

Do you have a dry mouth?

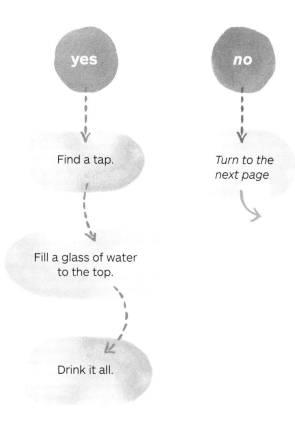

yes

Find a tap.

Fill a glass of water to the top.

Drink it all.

no

Turn to the next page

When people feel anxious, they often breathe through their mouth, which can reduce salivary flow. By standing up and taking the action of filling a glass of water, it can redirect our mind away from anxious feelings and, as a bonus, when we drink the water, our mouths are moistened.

Are you replaying
a scenario or conversation
over and over again
in your head?

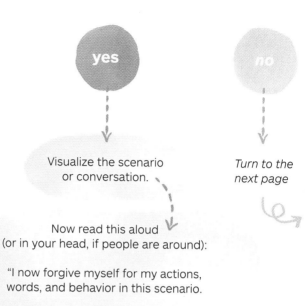

yes

no

Turn to the
next page

Visualize the scenario
or conversation.

Now read this aloud
(or in your head, if people are around):

"I now forgive myself for my actions,
words, and behavior in this scenario.

"I understand deep down that I did the best I could
with the resources and knowledge I had at the time.

"I have learned the lessons I need to,
so now I can move on. I can deal with
all ramifications of this event."

Inhale deeply.
Exhale all the overanalysis.

It is likely that you are ruminating. This is when your mind
repeatedly replays a situation you've been in, worsening
your mood and anxiety.

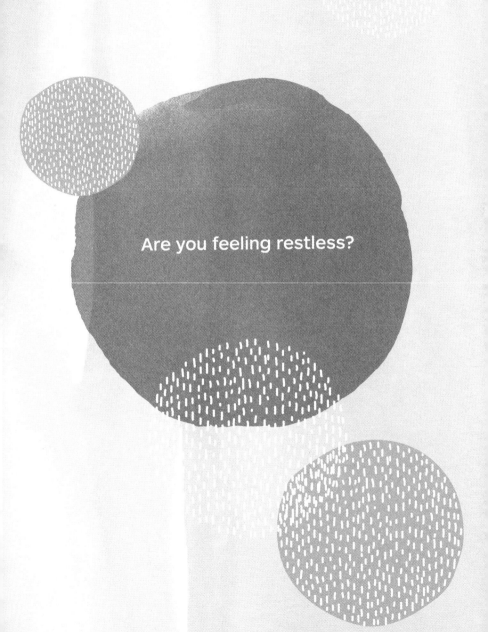

Are you feeling restless?

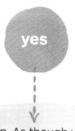

yes

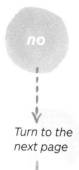

no

Stand up. As though you can "flick out" the agitation,

> Shake out your right leg
> Shake out your left leg
> Shake out your hips
> Shake out your right arm
> Shake out your left arm
> Shake out your head
> Shake out your whole body.

Turn to the next page

Bring to mind what you would like to focus on for the rest of the day.

Inhale deeply. Exhale all restlessness.

Take one immediate action toward your day's focus.

 When we have excess bottled-up energy, we can feel overstimulated, irritable, agitated, and restless. If we don't release that energy, we can end up distracting ourselves with unhelpful "fixes," such as food, alcohol, and TV. Regular exercise is one of the fastest ways to calm this feeling.

Are you procrastinating
or struggling to concentrate?

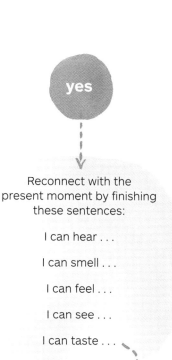

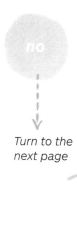

yes

no

Reconnect with the
present moment by finishing
these sentences:

I can hear . . .

I can smell . . .

I can feel . . .

I can see . . .

I can taste . . .

Turn to the next page

Still struggling to focus?

Write a list of all the
tasks you are avoiding.
Identify the least fun task
and start it right away.

Give the task
your full attention.

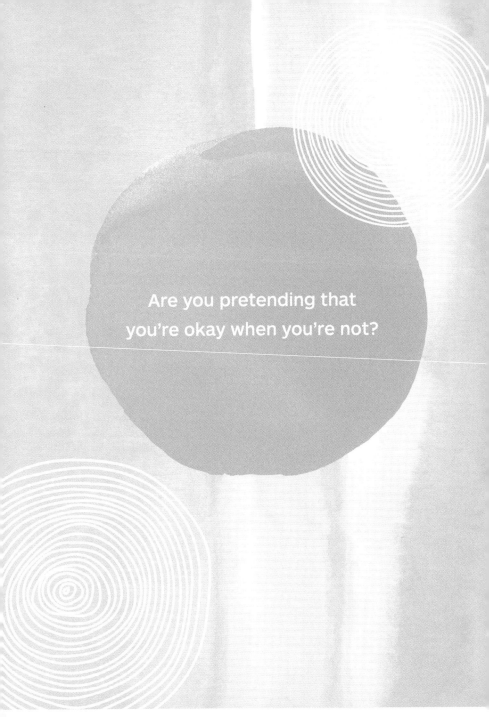

Are you pretending that you're okay when you're not?

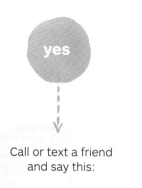 **yes**

 **no**

Call or text a friend
and say this:

*Turn to the
next page*

"Hi there, I wanted to reach
out to let you know that while I look
like I've got everything under control,
I've kind of been secretly struggling.
Can we catch up so you can
help me find a next step?"

 This is called masking. Masking is when we hide our real feelings,
often so we don't rock the boat or show vulnerability.

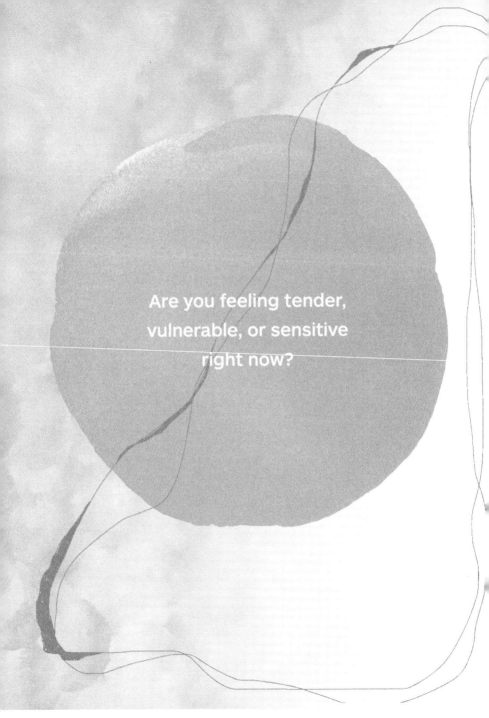

Are you feeling tender, vulnerable, or sensitive right now?

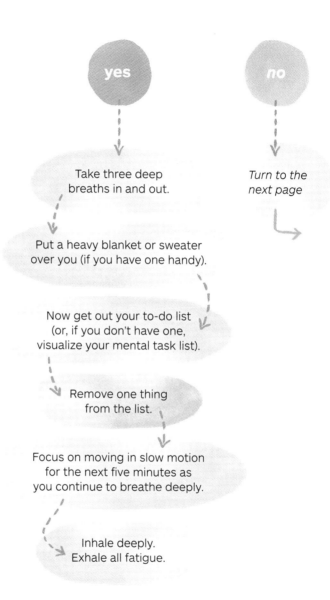

yes

no

Take three deep
breaths in and out.

*Turn to the
next page*

Put a heavy blanket or sweater
over you (if you have one handy).

Now get out your to-do list
(or, if you don't have one,
visualize your mental task list).

Remove one thing
from the list.

Focus on moving in slow motion
for the next five minutes as
you continue to breathe deeply.

Inhale deeply.
Exhale all fatigue.

Do you feel exhausted?

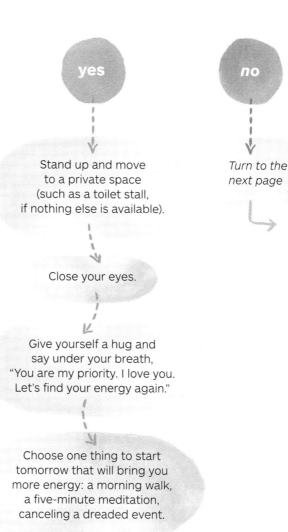

yes

no

Stand up and move
to a private space
(such as a toilet stall,
if nothing else is available).

*Turn to the
next page*

Close your eyes.

Give yourself a hug and
say under your breath,
"You are my priority. I love you.
Let's find your energy again."

Choose one thing to start
tomorrow that will bring you
more energy: a morning walk,
a five-minute meditation,
canceling a dreaded event.

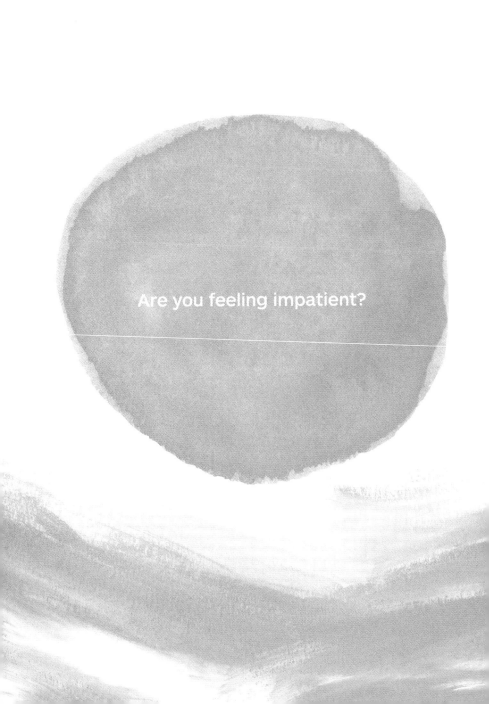

Are you feeling impatient?

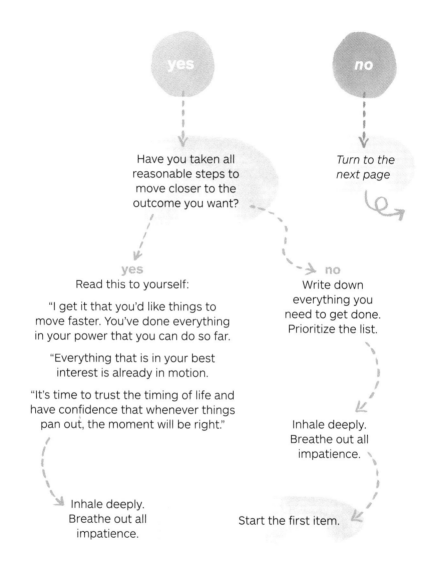

yes

no

Have you taken all
reasonable steps to
move closer to the
outcome you want?

*Turn to the
next page*

yes
Read this to yourself:

"I get it that you'd like things to
move faster. You've done everything
in your power that you can do so far.

"Everything that is in your best
interest is already in motion.

"It's time to trust the timing of life and
have confidence that whenever things
pan out, the moment will be right."

no
Write down
everything you
need to get done.
Prioritize the list.

Inhale deeply.
Breathe out all
impatience.

Inhale deeply.
Breathe out all
impatience.

Start the first item.

Is someone not reaching
your expectations?

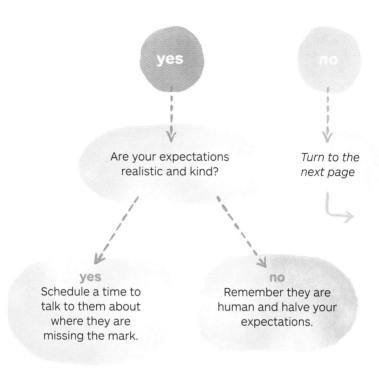

yes

no

Are your expectations
realistic and kind?

*Turn to the
next page*

yes
Schedule a time to
talk to them about
where they are
missing the mark.

no
Remember they are
human and halve your
expectations.

If you are in a relationship with this person and you need
further support, turn to page 87 to continue.

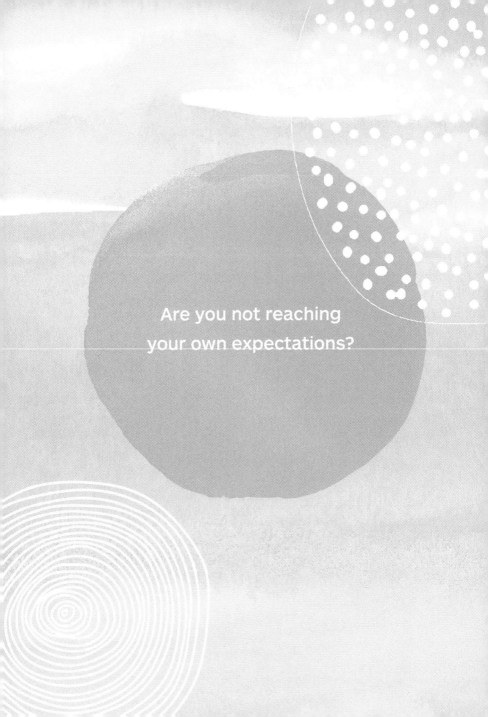

Are you not reaching
your own expectations?

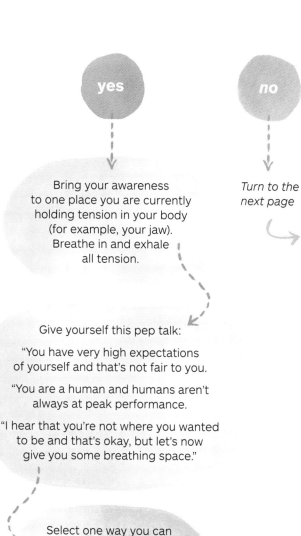

yes

no

Bring your awareness
to one place you are currently
holding tension in your body
(for example, your jaw).
Breathe in and exhale
all tension.

*Turn to the
next page*

Give yourself this pep talk:

"You have very high expectations
of yourself and that's not fair to you.

"You are a human and humans aren't
always at peak performance.

"I hear that you're not where you wanted
to be and that's okay, but let's now
give you some breathing space."

Select one way you can
lower those expectations;
for example, change
the time frame for
completion of a task.

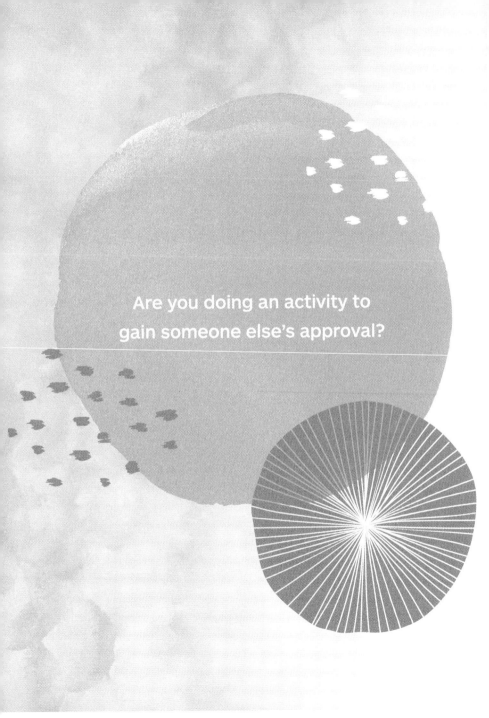

Are you doing an activity to gain someone else's approval?

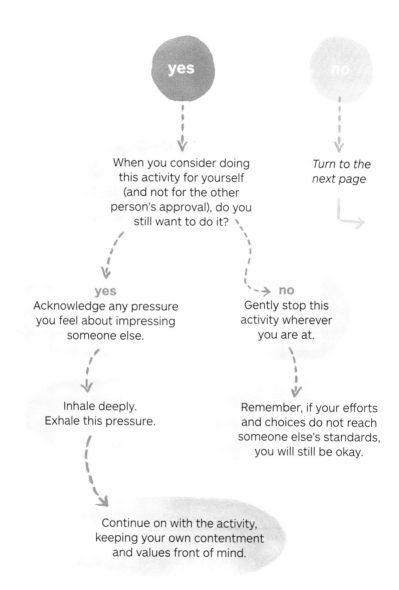

yes

no

When you consider doing this activity for yourself (and not for the other person's approval), do you still want to do it?

Turn to the next page

yes
Acknowledge any pressure you feel about impressing someone else.

no
Gently stop this activity wherever you are at.

Inhale deeply.
Exhale this pressure.

Remember, if your efforts and choices do not reach someone else's standards, you will still be okay.

Continue on with the activity, keeping your own contentment and values front of mind.

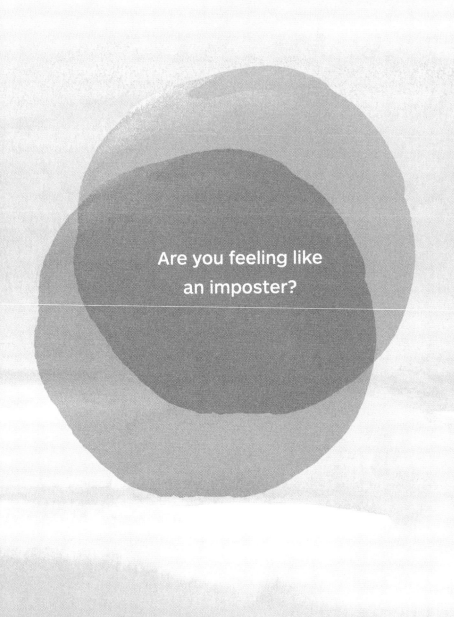

Are you feeling like
an imposter?

yes

Identify the scenario
that you're feeling
insecure about.

no

*Turn to the
next page*

Now ask yourself,
"Why do I deserve to . . . [insert your
identified scenario here; for example,
present to this group, be on this date,
be on this planet]?"

List five specific,
solid answers
to your question.

Inhale deeply.
Exhale all the fear.

"Imposter syndrome" is a non clinical diagnosis when an individual
feels like they're a fraud in their current situation, almost as
though they're going to be "found out." This can lead to feelings
of nervousness and anxiety.

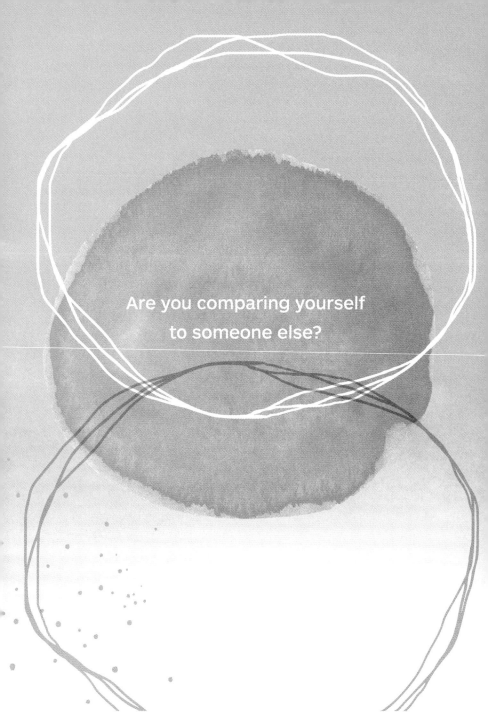

Are you comparing yourself
to someone else?

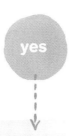 **yes**

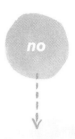 *no*

Bring to mind the person
you're comparing yourself to.

*Turn to the
next page*

Consider this concept:
If we judge others when they
have what we want, it pushes
our desire farther away.

Even if it feels tricky,
in your mind, say:

"Dear [their name], I'm so
happy for you for [insert milestone
here]; it's really wonderful.
Congratulations."

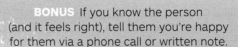

BONUS If you know the person
(and it feels right), tell them you're happy
for them via a phone call or written note.

Are you feeling run down?

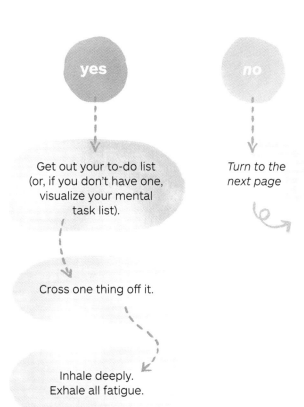

yes

Get out your to-do list
(or, if you don't have one,
visualize your mental
task list).

*Turn to the
next page*

Cross one thing off it.

Inhale deeply.
Exhale all fatigue.

no

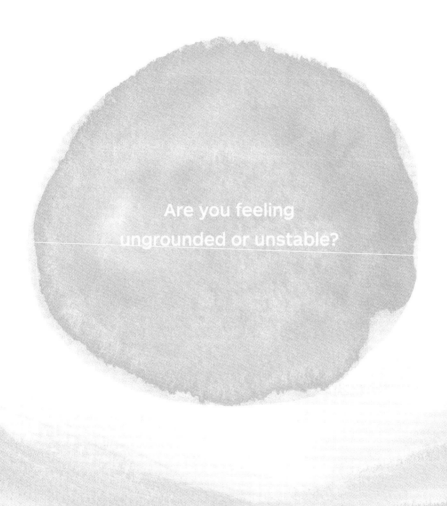

Are you feeling
ungrounded or unstable?

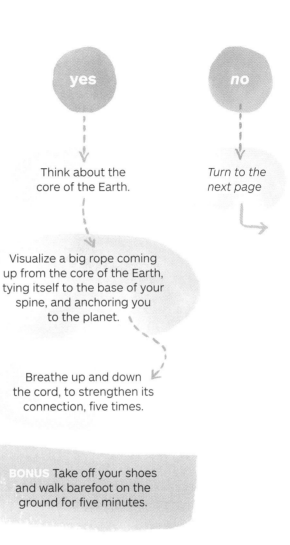

yes

no

Think about the
core of the Earth.

*Turn to the
next page*

Visualize a big rope coming
up from the core of the Earth,
tying itself to the base of your
spine, and anchoring you
to the planet.

Breathe up and down
the cord, to strengthen its
connection, five times.

BONUS Take off your shoes
and walk barefoot on the
ground for five minutes.

 When we lose connection with the Earth (and nature), it can lead
to feelings of disarray. "Earthing" or "grounding" is an important
component of our well-being.

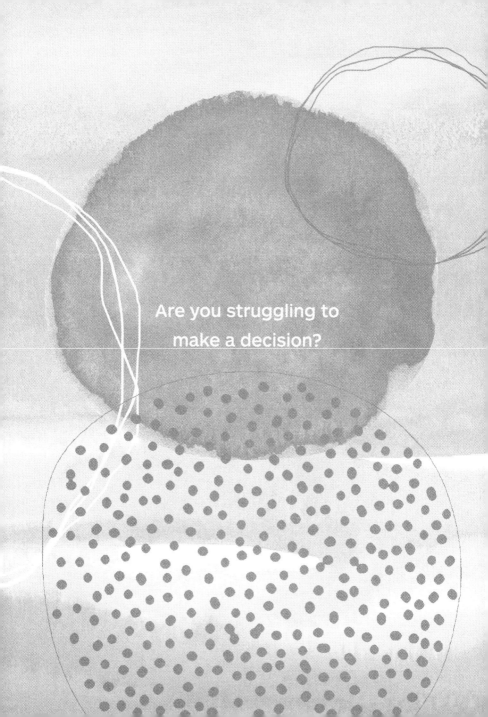

Are you struggling to
make a decision?

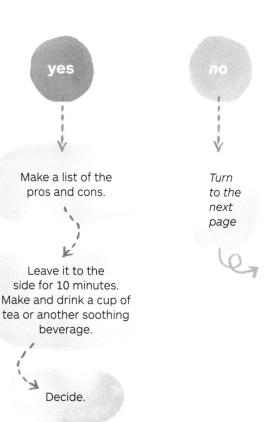

yes

Make a list of the
pros and cons.

Leave it to the
side for 10 minutes.
Make and drink a cup of
tea or another soothing
beverage.

Decide.

no

*Turn
to the
next
page*

Are you feeling teary
with the weight of other
people's emotions?

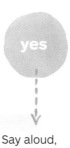

yes

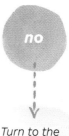

no

Say aloud,
"I now choose to breathe
out all emotions and feelings
that are not mine."

*Turn to the
next page*

Inhale deeply.
Exhale everyone else's
emotions and feelings
from your body.

If these emotions belong to your significant
other, turn to page 87, or if they belong to your
children, turn to page 107 for more support.

 People who are particularly empathic can sometimes unknowingly
take on the processing of other people's emotions. This sensitivity
can lead to feeling physically weighed down and can act as a
barrier to easy day-to-day functioning.

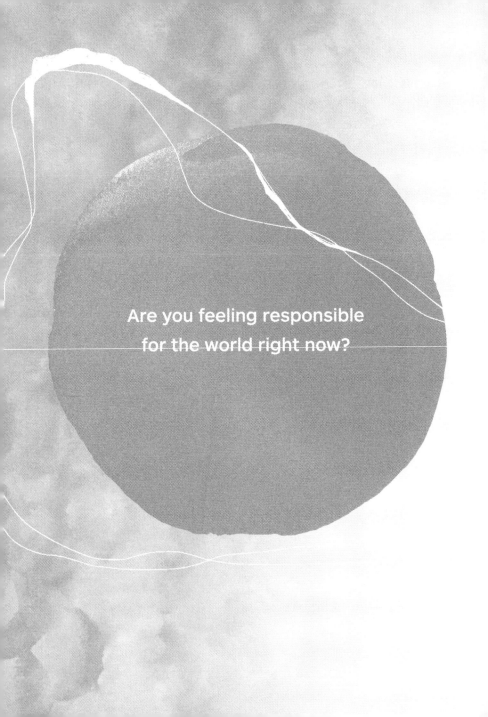

Are you feeling responsible
for the world right now?

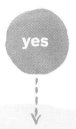

Read this to yourself
as though an older, wiser person
were speaking to you:

"It's not your job to save the planet.

"Today, your job is to breathe and
take good care of yourself.

"If tomorrow you still feel like making
a difference, you can take
one action at a time."

*Turn to the
next page*

Inhale deeply.
Exhale over responsibility.

This feeling might be due to an inclination to "fix" everything
around you. This is not your job, and trying to do it can lead
to inaction and reduced self-care. It is recommended that
any tendencies for "fixing" or "rescuing" others be replaced
by supporting them without attempting to solve problems on
their behalf.

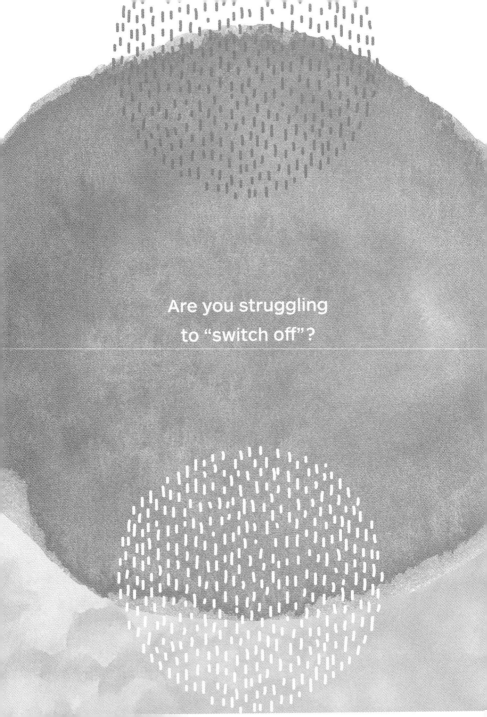

Are you struggling
to "switch off"?

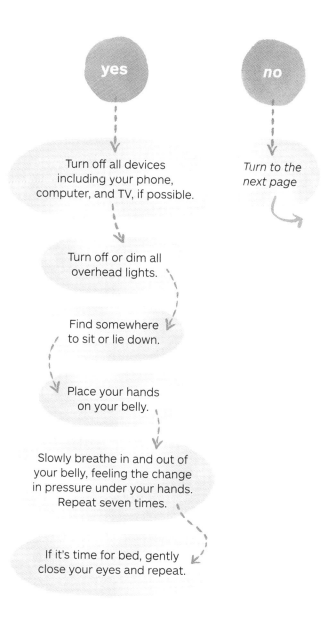

yes

no

Turn off all devices
including your phone,
computer, and TV, if possible.

*Turn to the
next page*

Turn off or dim all
overhead lights.

Find somewhere
to sit or lie down.

Place your hands
on your belly.

Slowly breathe in and out of
your belly, feeling the change
in pressure under your hands.
Repeat seven times.

If it's time for bed, gently
close your eyes and repeat.

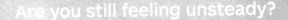

Are you still feeling unsteady?

If your unsteadiness relates to
social anxiety, turn to page 67.

If your unsteadiness relates to
your relationship, turn to page 87.

If your unsteadiness relates to
parenting, turn to page 107.

yes

no

Still not sure what your unsteadiness relates to?

You wonderful thing, you.

Even in the thick of worry and panic, you were able to move through this moment.

Tap repeatedly on the "karate chop" part of your hand.

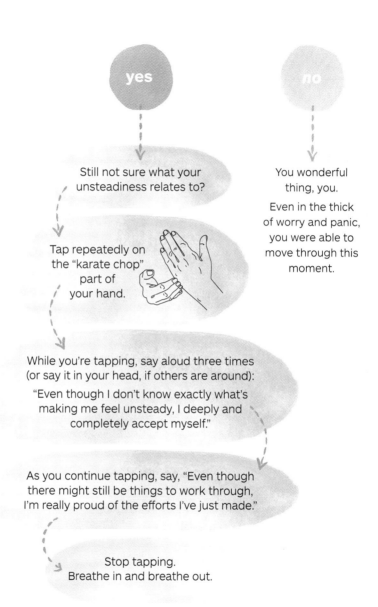

While you're tapping, say aloud three times (or say it in your head, if others are around):

"Even though I don't know exactly what's making me feel unsteady, I deeply and completely accept myself."

As you continue tapping, say, "Even though there might still be things to work through, I'm really proud of the efforts I've just made."

Stop tapping.
Breathe in and breathe out.

If you're experiencing anxiety related to:

> **Living & working** Turn to page 7

> **Relationships** Turn to page 87

> **Parenting** Turn to page 107

or read on . . .

Socializing

Interacting with others can be daunting.
Sometimes it can fill us with energy and at other times
it can deplete us. If you're currently worrying about
interacting with others or experiencing social anxiety,
turn the page to continue.

Are you nervous about
an upcoming situation where
you have to be social and
interact with others?

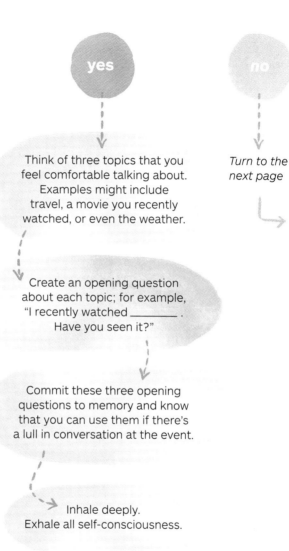

yes

no

Think of three topics that you feel comfortable talking about. Examples might include travel, a movie you recently watched, or even the weather.

Turn to the next page

Create an opening question about each topic; for example, "I recently watched _____ . Have you seen it?"

Commit these three opening questions to memory and know that you can use them if there's a lull in conversation at the event.

Inhale deeply. Exhale all self-consciousness.

Are you nervous about
an upcoming situation where
you need to "perform,"
such as giving a speech?

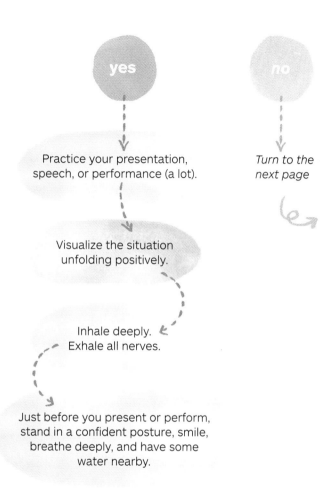

yes

no

Practice your presentation, speech, or performance (a lot).

Turn to the next page

Visualize the situation unfolding positively.

Inhale deeply.
Exhale all nerves.

Just before you present or perform, stand in a confident posture, smile, breathe deeply, and have some water nearby.

Are you
dreading
an upcoming
event?

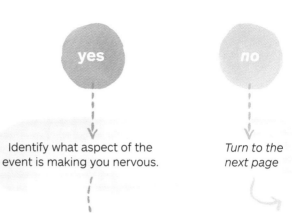

yes

no

Identify what aspect of the event is making you nervous.

Turn to the next page

Choose one small thing to do just before you enter the event that will help you feel more confident about that aspect.

Examples might include choosing to wear an outfit that makes you feel great or choosing to walk into the event with a confident posture.

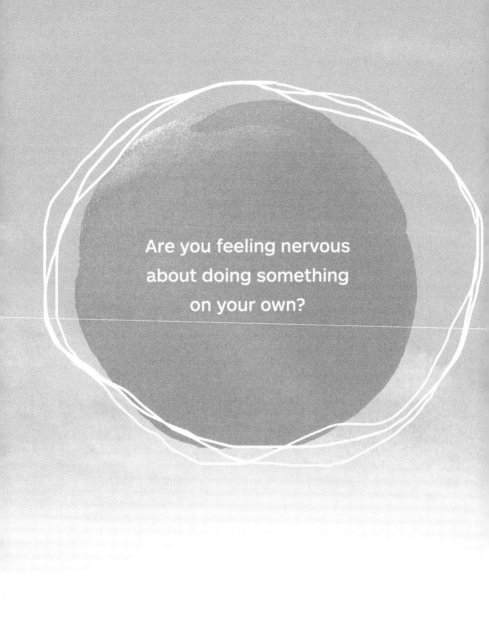

Are you feeling nervous
about doing something
on your own?

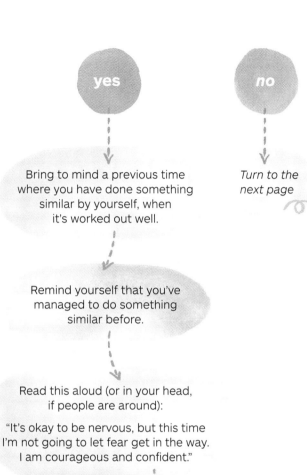

yes

no

Bring to mind a previous time where you have done something similar by yourself, when it's worked out well.

Turn to the next page

Remind yourself that you've managed to do something similar before.

Read this aloud (or in your head, if people are around):

"It's okay to be nervous, but this time I'm not going to let fear get in the way. I am courageous and confident."

Inhale courage.
Exhale nerves.

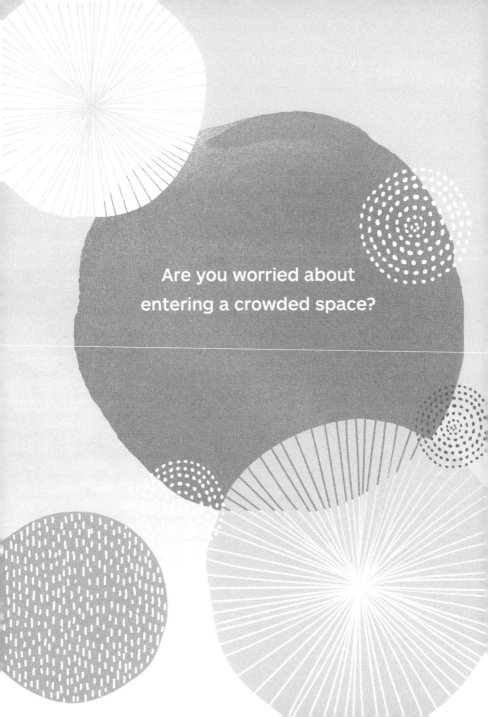

Are you worried about
entering a crowded space?

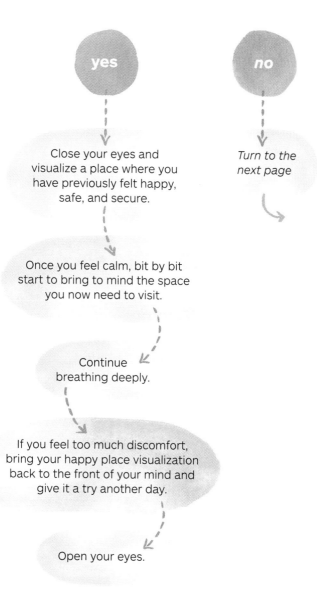

yes

Close your eyes and visualize a place where you have previously felt happy, safe, and secure.

Once you feel calm, bit by bit start to bring to mind the space you now need to visit.

Continue breathing deeply.

If you feel too much discomfort, bring your happy place visualization back to the front of your mind and give it a try another day.

Open your eyes.

no

Turn to the next page

Do you have a difficult
conversation coming up?

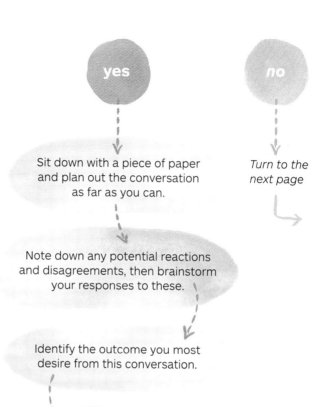

yes

no

Sit down with a piece of paper
and plan out the conversation
as far as you can.

*Turn to the
next page*

Note down any potential reactions
and disagreements, then brainstorm
your responses to these.

Identify the outcome you most
desire from this conversation.

Inhale deeply.
Exhale all apprehension.

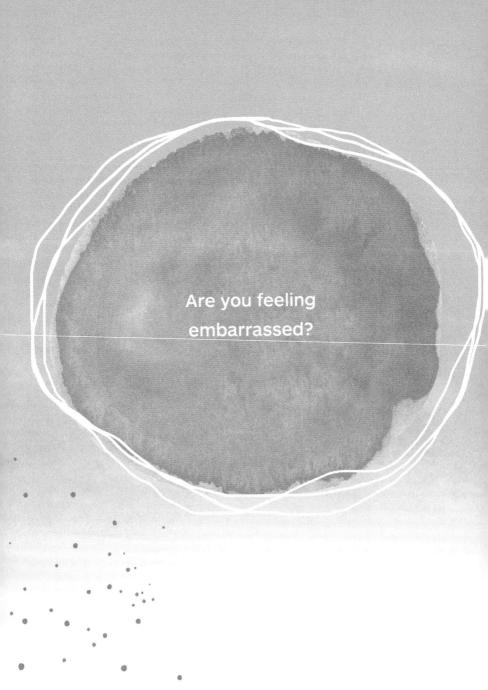

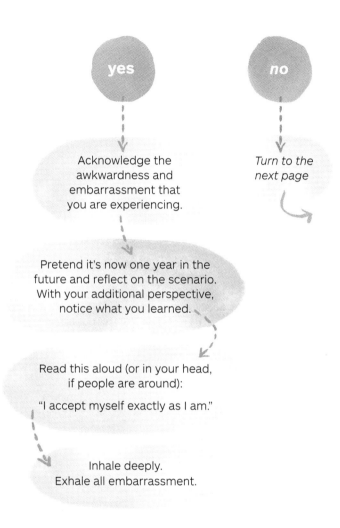

yes

no

Acknowledge the
awkwardness and
embarrassment that
you are experiencing.

*Turn to the
next page*

Pretend it's now one year in the
future and reflect on the scenario.
With your additional perspective,
notice what you learned.

Read this aloud (or in your head,
if people are around):

"I accept myself exactly as I am."

Inhale deeply.
Exhale all embarrassment.

Embarrassment is our brain's reaction to thinking we are being
perceived in a way we don't like and our heart's reaction to feeling
unacceptable in some way. It can be accompanied by blushing,
sweating, stammering, and fidgeting. Taking deep breaths can
help calm the physical symptoms.

Are you holding yourself
back from making new friends?

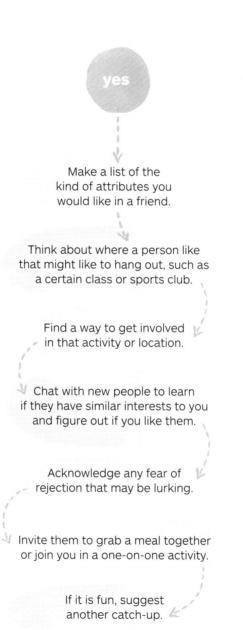

yes

no

Turn to the
next page

Make a list of the
kind of attributes you
would like in a friend.

Think about where a person like
that might like to hang out, such as
a certain class or sports club.

Find a way to get involved
in that activity or location.

Chat with new people to learn
if they have similar interests to you
and figure out if you like them.

Acknowledge any fear of
rejection that may be lurking.

Invite them to grab a meal together
or join you in a one-on-one activity.

If it is fun, suggest
another catch-up.

Are you struggling to ask for
help that you know you need?

yes

no

Identify exactly what type
of help you need.

You wonderful
thing, you.

Even in the thick
of worry and panic,
you were able to
move through this
moment.

Consider who has the skills
that can provide the answer
or support you need.

Decide what is the best way to
ask for help from them: in person,
by phone, text message,
or e-mail?

Use this method to
ask them for help.

If there is some uneasiness or worry still
hanging around, flip back to page 7 to help
neutralize any remaining anxiety.

Remember that asking for help is not a sign of weakness.
Asking for help is a sign of strength.

If you're experiencing anxiety related to:

> **Living & working** Turn to page 7

> **Socializing** Turn to page 67

> **Parenting** Turn to page 107

or read on . . .

Relationships

Relationships with a significant other can be tricky.
While they can bring huge amounts of joy, connection,
and togetherness, sometimes they wobble.
If you're currently experiencing worry about your
relationship, turn the page to continue.

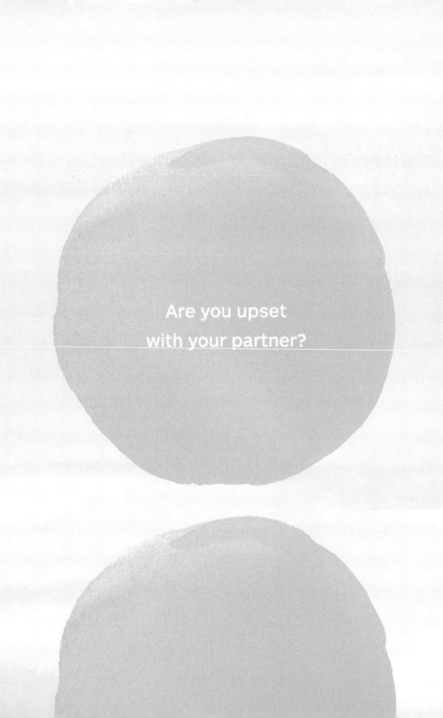

Are you upset
with your partner?

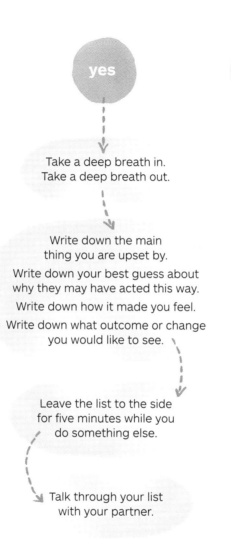

yes

Take a deep breath in.
Take a deep breath out.

Write down the main
thing you are upset by.

Write down your best guess about
why they may have acted this way.

Write down how it made you feel.

Write down what outcome or change
you would like to see.

Leave the list to the side
for five minutes while you
do something else.

Talk through your list
with your partner.

no

*Turn to the
next page*

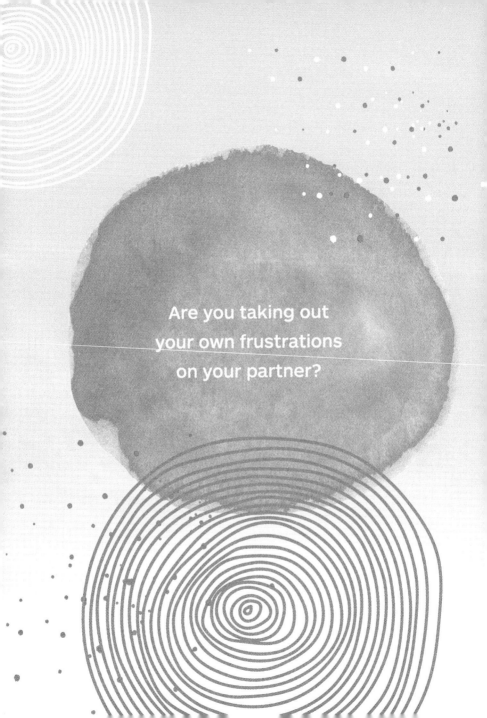

Are you taking out
your own frustrations
on your partner?

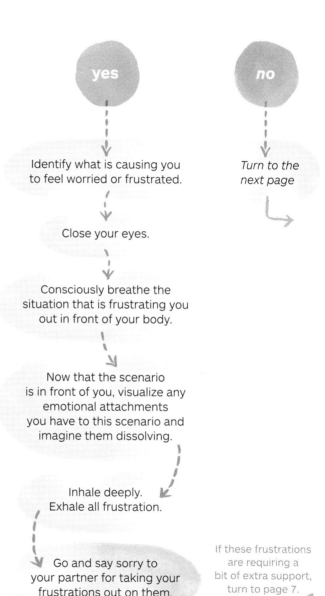

yes

Identify what is causing you to feel worried or frustrated.

Close your eyes.

Consciously breathe the situation that is frustrating you out in front of your body.

Now that the scenario is in front of you, visualize any emotional attachments you have to this scenario and imagine them dissolving.

Inhale deeply.
Exhale all frustration.

Go and say sorry to your partner for taking your frustrations out on them.

no

Turn to the next page

If these frustrations are requiring a bit of extra support, turn to page 7.

Has there been a
communication breakdown
between you and
your partner?

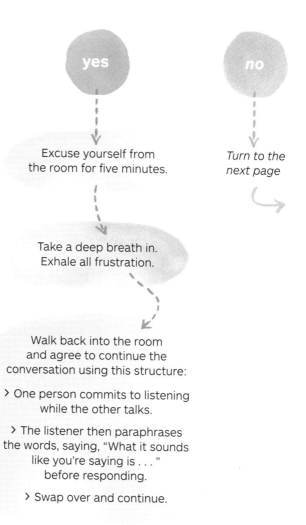

yes

no

Excuse yourself from
the room for five minutes.

*Turn to the
next page*

Take a deep breath in.
Exhale all frustration.

Walk back into the room
and agree to continue the
conversation using this structure:

> One person commits to listening
while the other talks.

> The listener then paraphrases
the words, saying, "What it sounds
like you're saying is . . . "
before responding.

> Swap over and continue.

Do you and your partner
have different standards
when it comes to housework/
ambition/money/other?

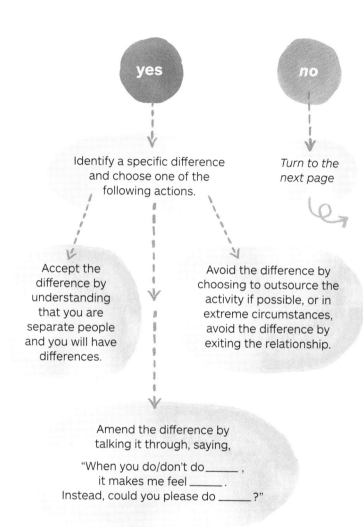

yes

Identify a specific difference and choose one of the following actions.

no

Turn to the next page

Accept the difference by understanding that you are separate people and you will have differences.

Avoid the difference by choosing to outsource the activity if possible, or in extreme circumstances, avoid the difference by exiting the relationship.

Amend the difference by talking it through, saying,

"When you do/don't do _____ ,
it makes me feel _____ .
Instead, could you please do _____ ?"

Does it feel like your partner is taking more than they're giving?

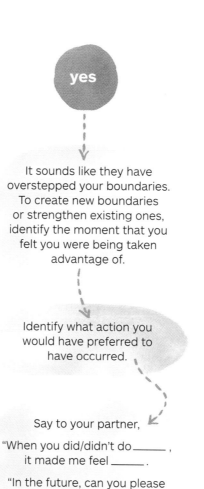

yes

no

It sounds like they have overstepped your boundaries. To create new boundaries or strengthen existing ones, identify the moment that you felt you were being taken advantage of.

Turn to the next page

Identify what action you would have preferred to have occurred.

Say to your partner,

"When you did/didn't do _____, it made me feel _____.

"In the future, can you please do _____instead?"

Are you worried that you're growing at a different rate to your partner?

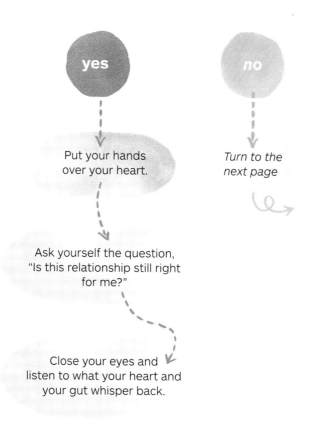

yes

no

Put your hands
over your heart.

*Turn to the
next page*

Ask yourself the question,
"Is this relationship still right
for me?"

Close your eyes and
listen to what your heart and
your gut whisper back.

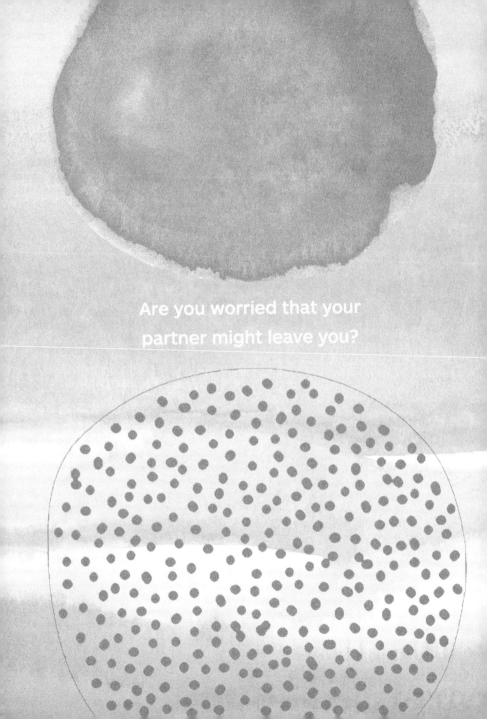

Are you worried that your
partner might leave you?

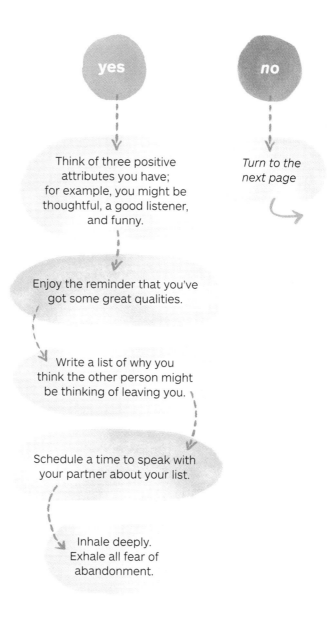

yes

no

Think of three positive
attributes you have;
for example, you might be
thoughtful, a good listener,
and funny.

*Turn to the
next page*

Enjoy the reminder that you've
got some great qualities.

Write a list of why you
think the other person might
be thinking of leaving you.

Schedule a time to speak with
your partner about your list.

Inhale deeply.
Exhale all fear of
abandonment.

Are you shy in the bedroom?

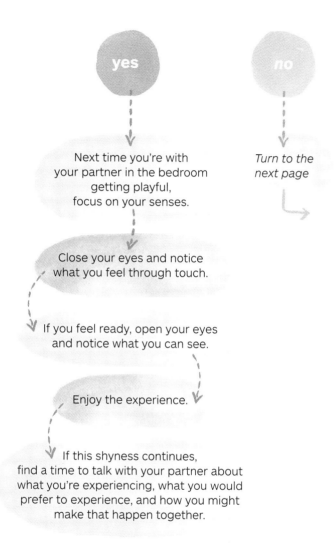

yes

no

Next time you're with
your partner in the bedroom
getting playful,
focus on your senses.

Turn to the
next page

Close your eyes and notice
what you feel through touch.

If you feel ready, open your eyes
and notice what you can see.

Enjoy the experience.

If this shyness continues,
find a time to talk with your partner about
what you're experiencing, what you would
prefer to experience, and how you might
make that happen together.

Sexual performance anxiety is closely linked with state of mind,
self-image, and confidence in the ability to please a partner.
When someone's mind is clouded with worry, it's difficult for
their body to get or stay "in the mood."

Do you feel numb about
your relationship right now?

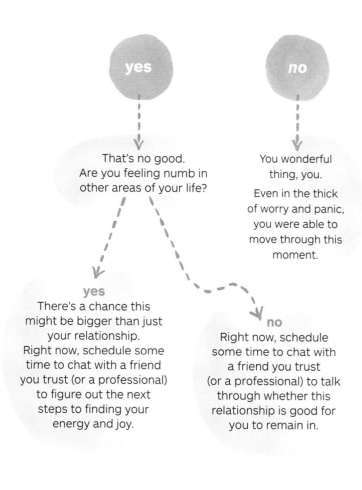

yes

That's no good.
Are you feeling numb in
other areas of your life?

no

You wonderful
thing, you.

Even in the thick
of worry and panic,
you were able to
move through this
moment.

yes

There's a chance this
might be bigger than just
your relationship.
Right now, schedule some
time to chat with a friend
you trust (or a professional)
to figure out the next
steps to finding your
energy and joy.

no

Right now, schedule
some time to chat with
a friend you trust
(or a professional) to talk
through whether this
relationship is good for
you to remain in.

If there is some uneasiness or worry still
hanging around, flip back to page 7 to help
neutralize any remaining anxiety.

If you're experiencing anxiety related to:

> Living & working Turn to page 7

> Socializing Turn to page 67

> Relationships Turn to page 87

or read on . . .

Parenting

Figuring out what to do as a parent while taking
care of yourself can be pretty tricky.
If you're currently experiencing worry relating
to parenting, turn the page to continue.

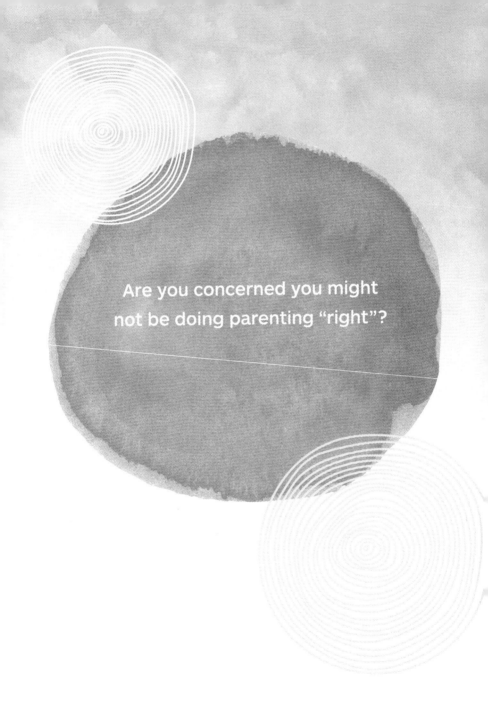

Are you concerned you might
not be doing parenting "right"?

yes

no

Remind yourself that there is no one "right" way to parent.

Turn to the next page

Get out a piece of paper.

Write down five things that you are doing really well as a parent.

Read your own list.

Breathe in the truth that you are doing the best you can. Exhale all doubts.

If these concerns about doing things "right" are broader than just parenting, turn to page 7.

Do you feel
bone-achingly tired?

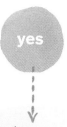

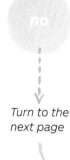

Imagine yourself
as a bank account.
Some people put in regular
deposits and other people put
in bits when they can.

For the short term,
you're the second person.
Whenever you get even a minute
of rest or sleep consider it
a deposit in the bank.

While it may not be the savings
plan you hoped for, know that
you're still making deposits.

*Turn to the
next page*

Inhale deeply.
Exhale all frustration with
your energy levels.

BONUS If you have the option
to capture more time to meditate
or sleep, take it!

Are you worried about how your kids
are progressing with their health/
developmental milestones/emotions/
social well-being?

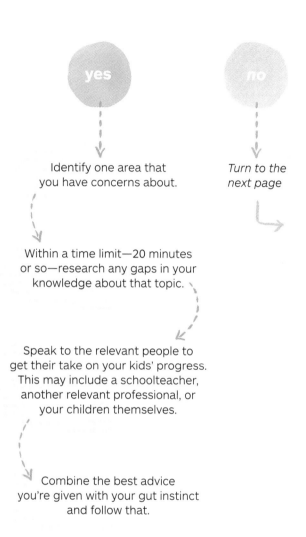

yes

no

Identify one area that
you have concerns about.

*Turn to the
next page*

Within a time limit—20 minutes
or so—research any gaps in your
knowledge about that topic.

Speak to the relevant people to
get their take on your kids' progress.
This may include a schoolteacher,
another relevant professional, or
your children themselves.

Combine the best advice
you're given with your gut instinct
and follow that.

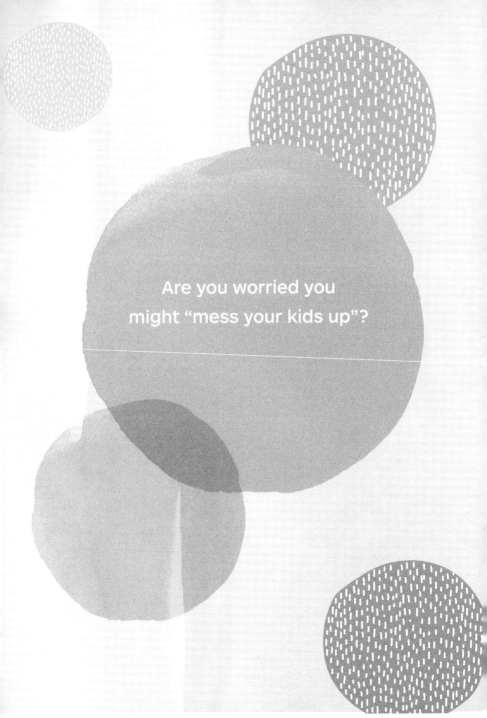

Are you worried you might "mess your kids up"?

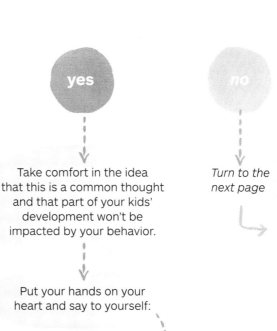

yes

no

Take comfort in the idea that this is a common thought and that part of your kids' development won't be impacted by your behavior.

Turn to the next page

Put your hands on your heart and say to yourself:

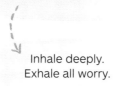

"Even though I'm doing my best, part of my children's development is out of my hands. They have their own minds and their own personalities, and I choose to honor that by doing my best and taking the pressure off myself to raise them perfectly."

Inhale deeply.
Exhale all worry.

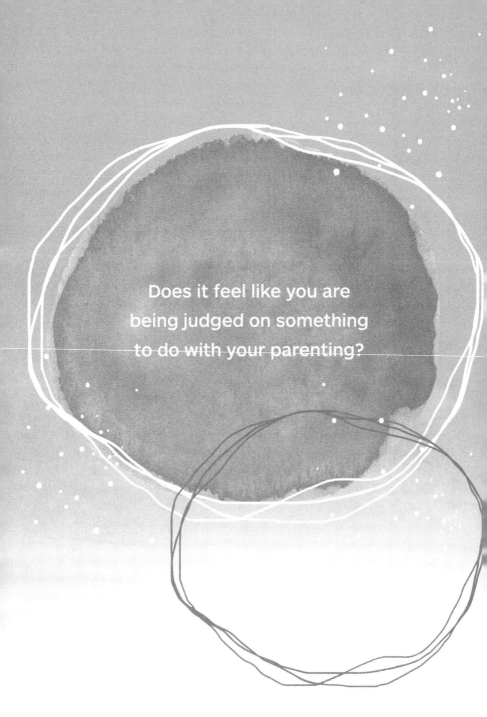

Does it feel like you are
being judged on something
to do with your parenting?

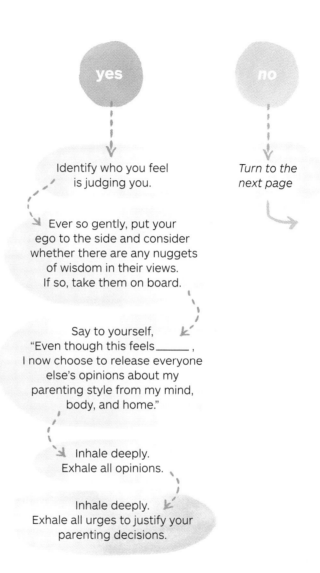

yes

no

Identify who you feel
is judging you.

*Turn to the
next page*

Ever so gently, put your
ego to the side and consider
whether there are any nuggets
of wisdom in their views.
If so, take them on board.

Say to yourself,
"Even though this feels_____ ,
I now choose to release everyone
else's opinions about my
parenting style from my mind,
body, and home."

Inhale deeply.
Exhale all opinions.

Inhale deeply.
Exhale all urges to justify your
parenting decisions.

When people judge others, it's often a silent way of justifying
decisions made in their own life. Although it may feel unpleasant,
remember that they are also doing their best right now.

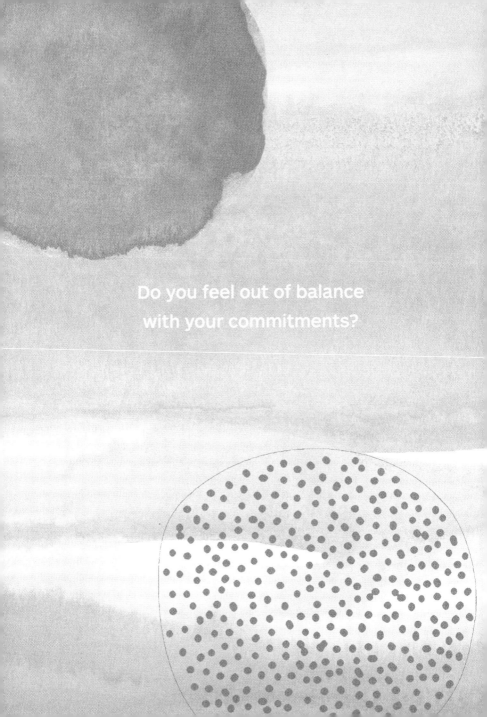

Do you feel out of balance
with your commitments?

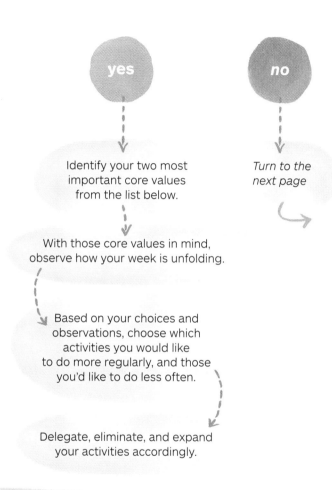

yes

Identify your two most
important core values
from the list below.

With those core values in mind,
observe how your week is unfolding.

Based on your choices and
observations, choose which
activities you would like
to do more regularly, and those
you'd like to do less often.

Delegate, eliminate, and expand
your activities accordingly.

no

*Turn to the
next page*

CORE VALUES Adventure · Authenticity · Business
Career · Community · Creativity · Energy · Faith · Family
Freedom · Happiness · Harmony · Health · Inclusion
Independence · Learning · Love · Respect
Security · Spirituality · Travel · Wealth

Are you craving your
pre-children lifestyle?

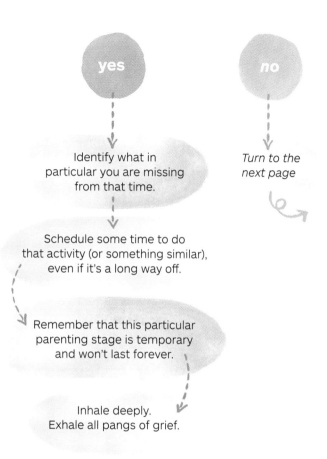

yes

no

Identify what in
particular you are missing
from that time.

Turn to the
next page

Schedule some time to do
that activity (or something similar),
even if it's a long way off.

Remember that this particular
parenting stage is temporary
and won't last forever.

Inhale deeply.
Exhale all pangs of grief.

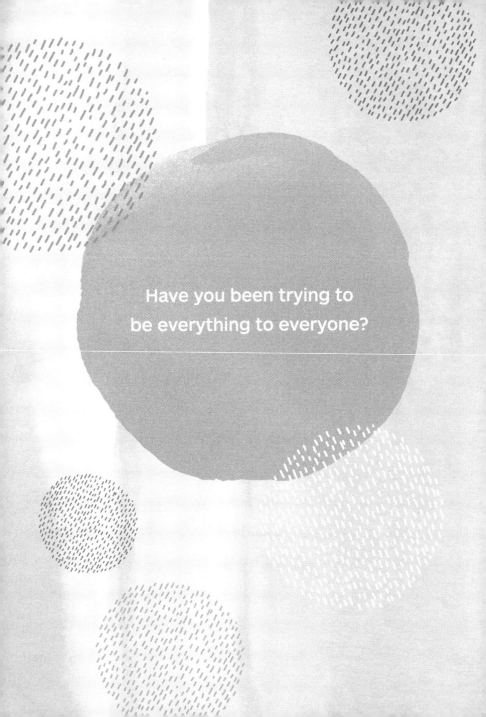

Have you been trying to
be everything to everyone?

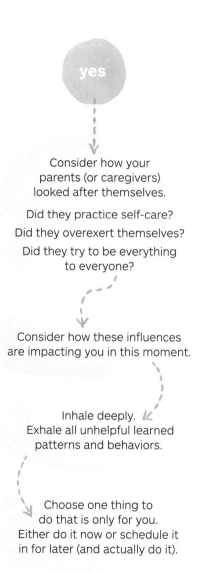

yes

Consider how your
parents (or caregivers)
looked after themselves.

Did they practice self-care?
Did they overexert themselves?
Did they try to be everything
to everyone?

Consider how these influences
are impacting you in this moment.

Inhale deeply.
Exhale all unhelpful learned
patterns and behaviors.

Choose one thing to
do that is only for you.
Either do it now or schedule it
in for later (and actually do it).

no

*Turn to the
next page*

Are you feeling unsupported
in taking care of your kids?

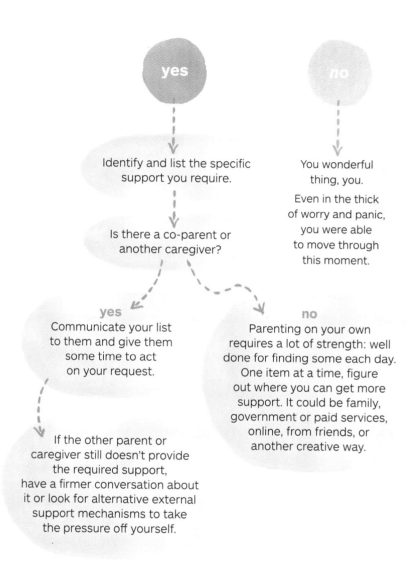

yes

Identify and list the specific support you require.

Is there a co-parent or another caregiver?

yes
Communicate your list to them and give them some time to act on your request.

If the other parent or caregiver still doesn't provide the required support, have a firmer conversation about it or look for alternative external support mechanisms to take the pressure off yourself.

no

You wonderful thing, you.

Even in the thick of worry and panic, you were able to move through this moment.

no
Parenting on your own requires a lot of strength: well done for finding some each day. One item at a time, figure out where you can get more support. It could be family, government or paid services, online, from friends, or another creative way.

If there is some uneasiness or worry still hanging around, flip back to page 7 to help neutralize any remaining anxiety.

Resources

Page 11: Box breathing was developed by former US Navy SEAL Mark Divine.

Page 65: The "karate chop" technique forms part of Emotional Freedom Techniques (EFT) practice, developed by Gary Craig.

Page 95: Inspired by the *AAAbc's of Stress*, developed by Nancy Loving Tubesing.

For emergency support, please contact your local helpline.

> The Lifeline (National Suicide Prevention Lifeline)
suicidepreventionlifeline.org
1-800-273-8255

> National Alliance on Mental Illness (NAMI)
nami.org
1-800-950-6264

> Anxiety and Depression Association of America (ADAA)
adaa.org
1-240-485-1001

> National Institute of Mental Health (NIMH)
nimh.nih.gov
1-866-615-6464

Acknowledgments

If you want to write a book (do it!), make sure you do your best to get a tribe of people as divine as mine to help make it happen. With intelligence and heart, Jane Morrow and the Murdoch Books team have helped craft, edit, design, and share this book. Empowered women really do empower other women.

They say you don't choose your family, but if I could, I'd choose mine. It is through their energy and strength that my path was initiated and shaped. Thanks to my mum, who reminds me that it's okay to take the pressure off myself, and always says that with a cup of tea, most things will feel better; to my dad, who shows me that logical rigor (hello, decision trees!) can be combined with a great depth of care and, when it is, amazing things are created; to my sister Trinette, who reminds me of the importance of quality time, and to my other sister Marnie, who helps me to see the beauty of the world through the eyes of an artist.

And finally, to the catalyst for this book, my handsome husband, Ivan: thank you for bringing lightness and safety to my days. You have given me the sanctuary to fall apart; just knowing this means it happens less.

P.S. To all the coaches, academics, spiritual teachers, yogis, psychologists, light workers, authors, and thought leaders who have helped pave the path for those of us who work holistically, thank you. Your perseverance in discovering new ways of helping those around you has helped me do the same.

Text copyright © 2020 by Tammi Kirkness

Design copyright © 2020 by Murdoch Books

First published in 2020 by Murdoch Books, an imprint of Allen & Unwin

All rights reserved

For information about permission to reproduce selections from
this book, write to trade.permissions@hmhco.com or to
Permissions, Houghton Mifflin Harcourt Publishing Company,
3 Park Avenue, 19th Floor, New York, New York 10016.

hmhbooks.com

Library of Congress Cataloging-in-Publication Data is available
ISBN 978-0-358-52594-3

Book design by Trisha Garner

Printed in the United States of America

DOC 10 9 8 7 6 5 4 3 2 1